HOW TO CURE

ECZEMA

How To Cure Eczema

Natural Eczema Treatment To Get Rid Of Skin Problems Once And For All

Alyssa Richards

TABLE OF CONTENT

What Is Eczema

Eczema is a condition which is often misunderstood by those who don't have it. Only those who have this condition would know how badly this condition can affect a person's life.

According to the dictionary, eczema is defined as 'an inflammatory condition of the skin, often characterized by redness, itching and oozing vesicular lesions which become scaly, crusted or hardened.'

The basic explanation of eczema may give you a rough understanding of the condition. This is an extremely uncomfortable condition to suffer from. However, it is even worse for someone who suffers as it not only impacts a person physically, but psychologically as well.

From this book, you would discover that eczema has a long history. It has impacted many people over thousands of years, but, there is still no solid cure for eczema. We have still continued to suffer from them.

Like most of the skin problems, eczema is a condition where most people try to treat on a superficial level. This is because our modern medicine tends to have this same attitude towards such problems.

However in this book, we would look to deal with eczema more naturally. Many of the solutions that you read in this book are more holistic in getting rid of simply minimizing the terrible effects of eczema.

On a topical level, there are many things that you could do to help reduce the severity of your problem. This is mostly done using natural substances.

In this book, you would find other methods which you can use to deal with eczema from the inside rather than just externally. Though, we would first look deeper at the eczema problem in the next few chapters before looking at the various treatments in dealing with your eczema problems.

Anyone Can Get Eczema

Question: What Exactly Is Eczema?

There is a great deal of mystery when it comes to this skin condition of eczema. Eczema refers to a set of clinical characteristics rather than one particular condition. As such, the definition of the causes of eczema is often unsystematic and hard to understand.

Throughout the years, there had been several terms and names which has been used to describe this condition from the experts and they have slowly come out with their own definition of what is eczema and what is not.

Because of this confusion, many people confuse this condition with psoriasis. However, these two conditions are not the same.

The difference between these two conditions is that eczema is normally found on the flexor aspect of body joints while psoriasis is not normally found in those areas. Generally, the flexor aspect of body joints refers to the body parts inside a joint which could decrease in size or surface while flexing.

Generally, it is agreed that eczema is a major form of dermatitis. Dermatitis is normally a term used as a catch-all for any sort of inflammation of the epidermis, which is known as the outer-most layer of the human skin. As such, many non-medical professionals would use the two words eczema and dermatitis almost identically. As such, you would hear that eczema is commonly referred to as dermatitis eczema. Very confusing huh!

If you are a laymen, you would find that all these information may confuse or overwhelm you. It may do nothing to give you a clearer picture on what eczema is. We all know that eczema is the inflammation of your skin, however, there is more to know than that.

Question: Who Would Normally Be Prone To Eczema?

Anyone!

Yes, anyone can suffer from eczema. Although it is a condition which most commonly starts when someone is a mere baby, it could strike anyone. It could impact men and women, regardless of age.

However, the effects of eczema would be different from people. Most commonly, eczema is normally characterized by having dry, red patches on your skin which are very itchy.

Unfortunately, as most people would have a tendency to scratch the itch, this makes it an even more difficult condition to deal with. Although some people may understand that they shouldn't scratch, they would still end up scratching. Eczema is sometimes known as the itch which causes rashes, because very often, the moment you scratch the itch, it would generate a rash.

In toddler and young children, eczema normally appears as dry patches which are red in color. This is found on the neck, scalp, forehead, forearms and legs. For most children, this condition would gradually slow down as they grow older. As such, many children who suffered from eczema when they were a baby or toddler would have no problems whatsoever when they become adults.

It should be known that there are many factors which triggers an eczema outbreak even when you are an adult. You may have cleared the condition for several years. When it happens to adults, the dry red skin would be most common around the elbows, knees but less on the ankles. At the same time however, this condition may flare up. This causes many of the childhood eczema characteristics to arise suddenly.

If you are in a chronic eczema condition, it should be clear that there isn't a clear cure for eczema although this condition isn't life threatening. There are various ways of treating the condition to ensure it doesn't flare up in the future. However, it should be noted that because most of the younger people are the group who commonly get eczema, they may find it hard to scratch. As such, they end up getting infections or other conditions which attack broken skin like warts.

Question: What Are The Different Types Of Eczema?

There are different types of eczema. Each of them is believed to have different causes. As such, the cause of it depends a lot on the particular condition that the eczema sufferer has suffered from. These are a few of the more common forms of eczema. I have also listed the most widely accepted causes of the different types of eczema. They include:

- **Atopic Eczema**

This is perhaps the most common form. It is believe to be hereditary and is something known as infantile eczema because of its hereditary nature. It is the form of eczema which is most common among children. If a parent suffers from eczema, hay fever or asthma; the child would have a significantly higher chance of developing eczema. As a matter of fact, if both parents have eczema, there is a probability of more than 80% that the children would develop eczema as well.

Researchers have found that if your child suffers from atopic eczema, their immune system is overreacting to certain external stimulus such as dust mites, pollen, animal hair or skin flakes. This leads to inflamed and irritable skin which is incredibly itchy. The child would exhibit most of the common eczema conditions mentioned earlier.

If the child scratches it often, it would cause the skin to bleed and raise a possibility of suffering from infection. Another problem that could arise is when eczema sufferers scratch their skin excessively until their skin becomes hard, tough or leathery. The lesions would dry out and this causes dry, flaky skin which is so common among those people who suffer from eczema flare-ups regularly.

Luckily, none of the atopic eczema suffering represents any sort of serious medical issue, although if the skin becomes broken and certain infections enter the body, the story would be very different.

However, any eczema sufferer would tell you that perhaps the itching is a symptom that could drive you nuts. Of course, adult sufferers would know better to not scratch, but it is easier said than done.

This condition is worse for children as it is very difficult to ask the child to simply stop scratching. Research has shown that scratching the itch does provide relief, although only temporarily.

Another common problem of atopic eczema is that there is a tendency in certain child patients to discharge a mixture of ear wax and mucus or even blood. This happens most commonly when the child has a certain eczema which happens on the surface or inside their ears.

This isn't something to be particularly concerned about as it isn't unusual. However, if blood is present, you should seek medical advice immediately so you could find out the cause of the problem.

As previously suggested, atopic eczema is a sort of condition which could aggravate by a weak immune system. Therefore, you should try building up your immune system to fight this condition.

Contact Dermatitis

This type of eczema happens when there is contact with irritants which causes an eczema flare-up. The reactions that you might face as a contact dermatitis sufferer may be one of two ways.

The first category is irritant contact dermatitis which is a type of condition that comes on very quickly once you are exposed to certain chemical substances which irritates your skin. Around three quarters of all contact dermatitis cases are irritant contact dermatitis.

This is commonly associated with the fact that this is the most common industrial diseased suffered by employees in many Western countries which are industrialized. This condition is heavily apparent in those people who work in heavy industries like iron smelting, chemical production and other sort of similar industries. They will suffer from contact dermatitis, even if the employee has had no past record or history of such problems in the family.

The second category of contact dermatitis is called the allergen contact dermatitis. This condition happens when the individual suffers from a delayed reaction to a previous contact to an allergy. This normally happens when in contact with ivy or pollen.

It should be noted that the two variation of contact dermatitis aren't mutually exclusive. This depends on the strength of a person's immune system. You could contact both forms of contact dermatitis at the same time if you have a weak immune system. If you are weaker, you might even develop atopic eczema.

Xerotic Eczema

This is an uncommon form of eczema which is caused when someone has seasonal dry skin which has become so dry and cracked that the tell-tale lesion starts to develop. This condition is more common among older people and the main areas that are affected are the limbs and torso.

The Cause Of Eczema

The cause of eczema is often... hereditary, as mentioned in the earlier chapters. It is perhaps the main cause of eczema. However, it has to be said that there are certain triggers which could cause a flare-up of the itchy red skin lesions which are commonly characterized by eczema.

A good example is that a flare-up of contact dermatitis would be brought about by something as innocent as wearing rough clothes like those made from wool or other rough fabrics. Additionally, there are certain chemicals which could trigger an eczema flare up especially in youngsters. This includes bleach, certain soaps, tobacco smoke and cosmetics.

Regardless, it has to be said that the most common cause of eczema is still hereditary. If one or both of the parents have suffered from an allergic reaction like asthma, there is a susceptibility that it would be passed on to the children.

One good example is that according to research, it is accepted that around 15% of people (including youngster and babies) may suffer from eczema. For around half of those children, their condition would improve over time. By the time they reach adulthood, they would be totally cleared from eczema.

However, not everyone is as fortunate. Some have to deal with this condition all their lives. Adult who have a persistent eczema problem in the United States amount to around 5% of the general adult population. This amounts to almost 18 million American people. As such, this statistic clearly shows the widespread commonalities of eczema.

A study also suggested that part of the reason for the eczema epidemic is because we have a modern obsession with detergents and soaps to ensure that we are clean. Another main reason to suggest that this condition has increased is because of the medical advancement. As such, there are more cases of eczema being brought to attention in recent years.

As there is so little known about this condition, there is similarly a lack of detailed knowledge about other things which could cause your eczema to flare-up. From many books to websites you read, you would know that the cause of a flare-up is different among different people. Therefore, it is very important to find out the cause of your eczema attack not merely from reading a book. You would need to find a doctor to perform a more thorough analysis of your condition.

However, there seems to be several factors which could cause the condition in those who suffer from it on a regular basis. As such, you can make the changes in your life that you need to ensure that you control the tendency of flare-ups. We will consider the most commonly cited causes of eczema as a method of investigating how you could deal with your eczema condition more naturally.

What You Eat

In the first chapter of the book, we have suggested that many doctors would deal with an eczema problem on a topical basis. From a point of view of treating it more naturally, it is often much better to treat this condition on a holistic basis. In another way, it is much better to deal with any medical condition from the inside out rather than from the outside in. Dealing with eczema is the same thing.

It is believed that many foods could actually exacerbate eczema. Therefore, it is recommended that you change your diet to remove the foods which are believed to bring about eczema or that could make your condition worse. Before you do so, it is important to understand that eczema is a condition which affects everyone differently.

There isn't any way you could know precisely what food would affect you. The saying that 'one man's meat is another man's poison' is definitely true. As such there is no way to know with 100% certainty in alleviating your eczema problem.

Generally, it is believed that many foods in the list could make your eczema even worse. As such, you would need to experiment. Try removing certain foods from your diet or your children's, if they suffer from eczema. Try until you have found out the food that affects your eczema flare-up.

You should try to remove certain foods from your diet or from your children's gradually. If you try to make drastic changes by stop taking a lot of food and see marked improvements, you wouldn't have any idea of what are the foodstuffs which were causing the problem previously. It may be frustrating for someone to change their diet or gain any meaningful insights from your 'diet change experiment'. However, try changing one thing at a time.

This process is often referred as the elimination diet - the process where you remove a particular group of foods from your diet and ensuring that you keep out the food group out of your diet for a certain period of time. Ideally, this should be for around two weeks.

During this period, try keeping a detailed diary so you could record on what is happening. If your eczema problem improves a lot by stopping certain foodstuffs but returns the moment you start eating them, you have isolated the diet problem which exacerbates your eczema.

Among the food groups that you should work on include:

Dairy Products: This is perhaps the first food group you should start with. This is the food group which is most commonly associated with causing eczema. Substances like milk or other foods which contain milk like yoghurt, cheese and ice cream can also cause eczema. It has been researched that processed foods should be or try to be avoided.

Generally speaking, there has been research being done that breast-fed babies are less likely to suffer from eczema from a baby who takes formula milk. If a mum is going to breast-feed, she should reduce the amount of dairy products she consumed during pregnancy. This is because what a mother eats or drinks would affect the nutrients that are present in the breast milk. This may cause eczema outbreak in the children.

Wheat-Based Products: Foods which contain wheat flour like biscuits, bread and pretzels are rich with gluten. Like many of the other foodstuffs you would find in this list, gluten can cause an eczema flare-up. As such, you should try removing them from your diet for a certain period.

It should be noted that beverages like coffee substitutes, root beer or beer may also contain grain and yeast. Yeast is a fungus which is another constituent of most bread products.

Fish And Seafood: Fish and seafood is another food group that you should try to eliminate and see whether it affects your flare up. Oily fish like tuna, salmon and sardine have all been found to cause eczema flare ups. Oily fish is generally accepted to be very good in helping you because it contains essential Omega-3 Fatty acids, but can be a problem for those who suffer from eczema.

However, it is hard to gauge what foods would cause an eczema sufferer problem. This is particularly true of Omega-3 fatty acids because it is found out that it could reduce inflammation in every part of the body rather than causing a problem.

Since eczema is a skin inflammation problem, it may be that some people could actually benefit from having it in their diet. Since this is so uncertain, you may want to try to include fish oil in your diet in order to increase the Omega-3 levels. However, be sure to keep a very close record of the results.

Besides that, it is also recommended that you use supplements rather than eating lots of oil fish. It has to be known that many predator oily fish, or those which get Omega-3 from eating other fishes, tend to eat a lot of toxins at the same time. For example, fishes like salmon and tuna have high content of mercury and dioxins. If you are someone who wants larger amounts of Omega-3 in your diet, use safe supplements.

It is also believed that in this same group, crustaceans like crab, prawns and lobsters may be the food that you should eat. As a matter of fact, it is still unclear is eating oily fish is good for someone with eczema problem. It cannot be a doubt that shellfish and crustaceans are common problem for people with eczema.

Eggs: Eggs or other food which are egg-based should be avoided. For example, food like cakes would often contain eggs. Egg allergies are very common. Some researchers suggest that being allergic to eggs or certain egg materials is a very common eczema problem among children.

However, to decide if you have a reaction towards eggs, you can simply perform an elimination diet. If you feel that eggs are causing a problem, test it out for a period of time. Stop taking them for a period of time and then reintroduce it in the future. If your eczema problems appear again, you would have a clearer picture of what causes problems.

Nuts: Nuts are a very common allergic problem among many people. 'True' nuts like pistachios, almonds, hazelnuts, cushion nuts and walnuts can make your eczema problem far worse if included in the diet. Peanuts are commonly believed to cause you more problems if you are someone with eczema, although peanuts are not even considered a nut. It is more of a legume, like peas or beans.

People who are commonly susceptible to peanuts as their cause of eczema have to check all the processed food in case for peanut traces. The practice of including peanuts traces in process food has decreased in recent years, but you still need to check for it. Make sure that there are no peanuts because the effects of it can be tremendous.

Acidic Fruits: There has been research which shown that acidic fruits like blueberries and cranberries could increase the probability of an eczema flare in many sufferers. Canned or glazed fruits would often cause a lot of problems as well because in the canning process, it is very common that they include artificial preservatives.

Food Preservatives Or Additives: Most of the more well-known food preservatives or additives can cause a flare-up. In modern day lifestyle, most of our foods include additives and preservatives to a certain extent. As much as you can, you should try to avoid food or drinks which are filled with chemical additives.

It should be noted that none of these chemical-based food additives are known natural. It goes without saying that if you want to completely ease your eczema problem, you should avoid food with preservatives or coloring in them.

Allergy Testing To Establish What Causes Eczema

In the past few chapters, we have shared that one of the most common causes of eczema is because of an allergic reaction. A person may be affected by certain allergens. We have also shared that many eczema sufferers are prone to allergic reactions to certain foodstuffs which prompt a flare-up condition at any time. The method of discovering what foods or drinks which cause eczema problems is through a journal of diet elimination.

This method has a great advantage that you could do anything at home and there isn't a need to spend money on anything other than a diary. However, there is another method of deciding what causes your eczema problem. This is to take an allergy test. This test would show you what exactly you are allergic to. It may take some time to see any substantial results as the allergist may have decided that there are different allergens you are allergic to. As such, the testing is a very slow process.

Besides that, an allergy test is also effective in deciding on any non-dietary factors which may cause your eczema. This includes an allergy to tobacco smoke, dust mites or even other form of chemicals like soaps.

Without a doubt, allergy testing is a more thorough method of deciding what exactly is causing your problem. As well as establishing allergies, this test would also establish a sufferer's individual personal reaction to various allergens.

However, it should be noted that allergy testing would only establish that the sufferer has a specific allergic antibody to the particular tested substance. It doesn't mean that an allergic reaction is the result of the presence of such antibodies.

As an example, an allergy test would establish that a person has antibodies which would react against substances like pet hair, but it doesn't follow that they would be automatically allergic or react to certain allergens.

Thus, if you are deciding to use allergy testing to decide the cause of your eczema condition, you need a test which could be interpreted by a qualified board certified allergist. When first starting to work with an allergist, they would ask you several questions about your lifestyle to establish the likely cause of your reactions to certain food or allergens. They may ask everything from your daily habits, family background or eating habits.

Generally, there are two kinds of allergy testing that are being accepted as scientifically valid. The first one is a skin test, which is the more preferred method of testing. In this situation, the tester would place a small drop of commercial prepared solution which contains allergen which the patient is assumed to be allergic on the skin before scratching the skin so the allergen enters the body.

When doing this, the allergist would look for a level of reaction from the patient to prove that they are sensitive to a certain allergen. However, as the initial allergen solution is considered too weak, it is very common that the allergist runs a few skin tests using a strong allergen solution in establishing the degree of adverse reaction which the patient would suffer.

The allergist is simply inducing an allergic disease artificially, in miniature. If the initial test on the skin isn't effective in deciding what the cause of certain negative reaction is, another similar test would be run by injecting the allergen solution under the skin.

The other form of allergy testing is known as the RAST (Radio-Allergo-Sorbent Testing). It is a kind of test to decide on the specific allergies antibodies in the blood and is a test which is improving in accuracy. It should be noted however, that RAST is more expensive than skin testing and the results often take a few days or weeks to arrive. As such, skin testing is still way more popular than RAST.

From performing an allergy testing, you would be able to have a clearer picture of the reason of your eczema condition. With this information, it becomes much easier to make the changes you need in your life to reduce your vulnerability to eczema.

Medical Treatments

To be diagnosed as clinical eczema, it is most commonly based on the patient's skin condition, family and personal history. These are all factors that decide if a person has clinical eczema. Besides that, there are also similar conditions to eczema and the medical practitioner would need to examine your skin lesions to decide on the real problem. They may carry out a skin lesion biopsy to decide on the exact condition you are suffering from.

Once the practitioners have decided that you are indeed suffering from eczema, they would recommend certain treatment dependent on the severity of the condition. Regardless of the treatment they decide for you, there would be certain common objectives of the treatment like:

- Clear any infection
- Reduce skin inflammation
- Controlling and reducing itching
- Loosen and remove scaly skin lesions
- Reduce outbreak of potential new lesions

There are several strategies which your medical practitioner would recommend as a way to use certain treatment in reducing the seriousness of the problem. This varies from applying topical pharmaceuticals, moisturizing your skin or other oral medications.

Very common, the medications which are being prescribed for the treatment of eczema are most probably based on corticosteroids. Corticosteroids are a type of steroid hormones which are naturally produced from the adrenal cortex.

Most medical practitioners would first recommend a topical cream or ointment, which are corticosteroids. This is the first-line of treatment. Many of those corticosteroid creams could be easily bought over the counter without prescription in most Western countries. The main reason for this is because the creams are not that strong. Their effectiveness is thus limited but the benefits are that it would unlikely to have any bad side-effects either.

Should your condition gets worse or doesn't improve at all, the doctor would prescribe a corticosteroid lotion or cream, which means that this treatment is considered much stronger than those you buy across the counter.

Besides that, it has been widely accepted by specialists that using corticosteroids over the long term could have terrible side-effects like irreversible skin thinning. As such, if you use such lotions or creams, only use them for a short period of time.

The third options which your medical practitioners recommend are oral corticosteroid drugs like prednisolone or prednisone. There are potential adverse side effects to these drugs and they are dependent on the strength of the drug you are taking as well as the period which you are taking them for.

Among the potential side-effects include high blood pressure, worsening of diabetes, weight gain, growth retardation in children and potential psychic disturbances.

It is fair to say that it is only in most serious circumstances that medical practitioners would prescribe the long-term use of corticosteroid drugs like these. Therefore, this treatment is very rarely prescribed by doctors.

As such, if you are prescribed with such treatments, you would need to take it with care. Your doctor may also prescribe antibiotics if you are in a situation where you have an infection due to the scratching of your eczema.

If you do indeed suffer from itching from your eczema, you may also choose to use antihistamines to reduce the seriousness. Antihistamine-based products are available both by prescription and across the counter. If you do decide to use antihistamines, you need to be aware that there are effects of causing drowsiness. As such, you should take this at night before you sleep. Don't ever take them if you are driving or before work as it can cause you to sleep.

The FDA approved two new drugs a few years ago which are known in the class of calcineurin inhibitors. These are drugs which would suppress the activity of your immune system to reduce the worst effects of eczema. Two most common types of drugs of this nature include Tacrolimus (Protopic) and Pimecrolimus (Elidel). However, it should be noted that there aren't many scientific evidence about any potential side-effects from taking this medication.

According to research however, if you avoid such medication, it would help the kidneys of renal transplant patient function more effectively and this points to a potential side-effect. Besides that, applying these drugs on your skin may also cause burning and discomfort for a couple of days.

However, less common side effects like acne, headaches and potential flu-like symptoms could also happen. As a matter of fact, the FDA has also issued a warning about a link between topically applied calcineurin inhibitors and cancer.

It could be clear from this chapter that medical practitioners are able to recommend many chemical-based pharmaceutical treatments when dealing with eczema. However, you may not want to use them as there are potential adverse side-effects from using them.

Since most eczema sufferers have a recurrent problem that isn't that serious apart from an irritating itch, even doctors are happier in recommending natural treatments to deal with the problem before using pharmaceuticals. In the next chapter, we would consider several natural options.

Dealing With Eczema Naturally

If you are someone who suffers from a mild bout of eczema, it is easy to minimize the effects of eczema to a more acceptable level with some home-based treatments. They are practical and effective.

For example, the moment you have found that the reason for your eczema flare-up is because of an exposure to a certain food, you should avoid putting yourself in a position of risk. The moment you know that seafood are the one that cause the problem, all you have to do is simply avoid eating them altogether. If your allergen is flower buds, then stay at home during the height of spring. As simple as that.

Since eczema is a condition which is characterized by having dry skin. It is very logical that anything which reduces your dry skin would be an effective method of dealing with your problem. As such, you should make sure that you don't bathe for too long while also reducing the amount of soap that you use. It is also better that you use natural moisturizing oil like tea tree oil as it ensures that your skin is moist and supple.

The moment you are out of your bath, it is important that you try to ensure that your skin is as moist as possible. This can be done by applying natural moisturizers like olive or tea tree oil on the dry areas of your skin. For best effects, do this within three minutes of you getting out of your bath as doing so ensures that you are applying moisturizer to your skin while it is still moist and flexible.

To increase the benefits of this strategy, it is helpful to wrap and dry the skin areas which you have applied those moisturizers with a plastic bag. This is to prevent your skin from drying out for the maximum period of time. Perhaps the main advantage of using olive or tea tree oil as a moisturizer is that they are very easy to find.

Like most aspects when it comes to dealing with eczema, there are certain contents of a moisturizer which is incredibly effective for most sufferers; however, they might not be suitable for you. As such, you may want to consider other alternative moisturizer made from substances which are completely natural:

- **Vinca Minor**: This is a type of homoeopathic moisturizing solution which is very effective in helping the sufferer to relieve sore, itchy and sensitive skin.

Therefore, it is ideal for someone who suffers from eczema to use moisturizer because dry and itchy skin is perhaps the most common characteristic of someone suffering from eczema.

- **Vitamin E Oil**: This is popular as it has the ability to hydrate the skin and promote healing at the very same time. This kind of oil helps to protect cell membranes while also promoting the ability of the body to use Vitamin K and selenium. As it has antioxidant qualities, it provides extra protection for your skin.

- **Calendula**: This is an ancient medicinal herb which helps treat dry and damaged skin. It is also powerful in minimizing the eczema effects and psoriasis. When used topically, this herb is effective in reducing your skin inflammation while also soothing irritated tissue. You can find plenty of places where you can buy the plants or the extract so you can make your own soothing, moisturizing lotion or oil yourself. If you can't find it, then only buy a commercial produced calendula salve.

The most important thing from this list is that the more regularly you moisturize the affected areas on your skin, the less problem that you would likely have.

As such, whenever you have washes away layers of moisture on your skin by showering, you need to replace it each time.

Another very common cause of eczema that you should try to avoid is to have extremes of heat or cold.

Although this depends a lot on the place you are staying, it is still a fact that many sufferers find it hard when they are in these extremes of temperature. By avoiding such extremes, you remove another potential cause of an eczema breakout.

Dealing With Stress

It is a common fact that those who are constantly stressed out or tensioned are more likely to exacerbate any chronic medical conditions that they have. Eczema is of no exception. When the sufferer has allowed their emotions to get to them, they end up being stressed up and the eczema would flare up. If you could reduce the levels of stress in your life, you would give yourself a better chance of avoiding outbreaks of eczema.

The very first thing you could do to reduce the stress on a daily basis is to simply change your life so you don't put yourself in stressful situations. If you are the kind of person who normally ends up running late each morning, try to get out of bed earlier (at least 15 minutes) so you have the time to catch the train so that you aren't that stressed every day.

If you are someone who has to rush to eat because you stay around your office during the break time, try to get away for half an hour to an hour so you can take a break from your work environment. Try finding for a place which is relaxed and peaceful like the part.

Besides that, you can also plan your meals at home in advance. As you do so, you ensure that you don't spend your evening after office rushing to the mall or convenience store to find food for your family.

If you are someone who is always at the beck and call of your family, try having some time for yourself. Perhaps some time to relax and pamper yourself. While it is great to be important to your family, you must realize that always being busy is something which is only going to damage your health. If you are constantly being there for them and you get sick, how are you going to take care for them?

The thing about stress is that it would normally flood your body with 'flight or fight' chemicals. This isn't entirely a bad thing, as it can be very helpful in certain emergency situations. However, if this becomes something constant in your life, it would only wear you down over time and causes further damage on your immune system.

If you start to slow down your everyday lifestyle, you would reduce the levels of stress. As you do this, the difficulties exacerbated by stress become less problematic for you.

As such, you need to really look at how you deal with the many areas of your life. If you find yourself being too stressed, you need to learn to cope with it. Give yourself time to step back to reassess the things that you are doing on your daily life. It is only when you know what you are doing that you can start changing it.

One great way is to keep a daily journal to see what you place as a priority. Try removing the inessential things in your life. With this information, you can start making change in your life to reduce daily stress in your life.

With addition to modifying your everyday lifestyle to reduce the stress amount in your life that exacerbates your eczema problem, there are also other things which you can earn to help you de-stress even more. One of the main practices that I recommend is yoga and meditation.

To start out with practices like yoga, it is normal to have to head out for organized classes which costs tremendous amount of money. However, it is now very possible to get most of this information from the internet. It is very well worth doing because yoga has a long history of being used for relaxation. It also helps as an exercise activity to build strength.

To obtain such information about how to start learning to relax using yoga, all you need to do is simply Google a term like 'how to learn yoga'. You would have tremendous amount of resources online. So you can learn everything you need to know from the comfort of your own home.

However, if you are looking to find resources faster and don't mind paying a small amount, you can easily head to website.

http://yoga.wellbeingvalley.com/

Besides using yoga, you can also combine it with other practices for slowing down your life and reducing stress. This includes learning to meditate, how to breathe deeply and even walking in the park. By doing this, you build your own relaxation routine to calm yourself down.

Practicing yoga shouldn't be focused on being an expert yogi, unless you want to. The main purpose is to train yourself to be relaxed daily. You have to find a practice which suits you. Give it a try and see how it would be able to change your life.

Eating Right To Cure Eczema

In the earlier chapters, I have shown you several foods and drinks that you should avoid. These foods or beverages may cause your condition to flare up if you are someone who suffers from eczema.

At the other side of the food argument, it should be noted that there are also plenty of nutrients that you should include in your diet to minimize the various unpleasant effects of eczema. You have to ensure that you have a diet which is rich in various nutrients to fight against eczema.

There are also other nutrient groups which has various other benefits from people suffering from eczema. This includes:

Vitamin B: It was one time believed that there was only a single form of vitamin B. However, it is now known that there are eight vitamins which make up the vitamin B complex.

The different forms of vitamin B have their own health qualities and they also work together as a team to help with various aspects of your health. The individual components of the vitamin B complex work with each other to ensure that the body functions in different way.

It has to be known that vitamin B complex could help boost the metabolic function and to promote muscle tone and a healthier skin.

Besides that, vitamin B also helps to promote a healthier nervous and immune system. It also helps promote cellular rejuvenation, cellular division and cellular growth.

Without a doubt, including vitamin B complex in your diet would help your skin and aid your immune system by protecting your body so it could fight back against eczema more effectively. There are several foodstuffs which are rich with various vitamins that make up the vitamin B complex. This includes food like green vegetables, potatoes, lentils and bananas.

Vitamin B can also be found in food like dairy products and eggs. However, there could also affect your eczema situation, as mentioned earlier in the chapter. Another alternative is to use supplements with vitamin B to increase the amount of this vitamin that you take in each day.

However, priority would be on eating actual food. If you find yourself struggling to eat such food however, you can go for vitamin B supplements.

Zinc: Zinc is a mineral which we all need in our diet because zinc has powerful antioxidant qualities. This would help prevent damage to your skin. It also helps stop the aging on your skin. Certain foods provide a great quality amount of zinc.

These foods include dates, roasted pumpkin, roast beef and squash seeds. However, the main problem with taking zinc in your diet is that most foods that are rich with zinc are food that you should be avoiding in the very first place. As such, zinc supplements are a better alternative.

Grape Or Cherry Juice: These juices have anti-inflammatory and antioxidant qualities. By drinking a glass of juice each day, you would give your body a boost in fighting against eczema better.

Fish Oil: Fish oil is very important in the fight of eczema as it contain Omega-3 fatty acids. This nutrient has various health benefits.

Fish oil also has a rich source of vitamin A, which has the qualities of maintaining a healthy skin while providing anti-inflammatory benefits as well. Note that eczema is a condition of your skin being inflamed. As such, sufficient amount of vitamin A is very important.

Cure Eczema From The Inside

From multiple researches throughout the years, it can be concluded one of the main reasons behind eczema is caused by an immune system which isn't strong enough. As such, using natural treatments or herbs to strengthen your immune system ensures that you are able to keep your eczema under control.

There are various herbs that are capable in improving your immune system's performance. This makes your ability to fight eczema from the inside better. As you start to include these herbs in your diet or supplementing them in your diet, you would slowly increase the chances of dealing with your eczema in a more holistic method.

In this chapter, I would share various methods of using natural herbs to boost your immune system. Some of these herbs, you may not have even heard of.

St John's Wort (Hypericum Perforatum)

This is a kind of plant which contains several compounds as it has a great number of well-documented beneficial psychological and medical effects.

St John's Wort is most commonly known as an antidepressant that is as powerful as pharmaceutical antidepressants. This is also a herb that has tremendous benefits for those sufferers of eczema as well.

You also have to understand that the ability to deal with mood swings or depression is very important. If this herb has the ability to deal with depression, it becomes less likely that you would suffer from any stress-related issues which make your eczema problem even worse. The most obvious benefits of St John's Wort however, is that it is a powerful anti-viral and antibacterial agent. This helps to boost your immune system's strength.

St John's Wort is also very effective in promoting a rapid recovery on your skin damage. Studies have shown that by applying them, it would help to recover burn trauma. This is especially beneficial for those people who suffered from burns. It has been proven that this herb cure burns up to three times faster than other pharmaceutical medications.

Sage (Salvia Officinalis)

This common sage which is incredibly effective in dealing with skin conditions like eczema is commonly referred to topical skin applications that are soothing and reviving. This herb is one of the best herbs in dealing with the eczema problem.

Sage is packed with powerful antioxidants and it is very effective in dealing with eczema. Besides that, it also has antibacterial qualities and is known as a stimulant for your immune system.

The most common benefit of using sage both as an herbal-based eczema component for topical use and using them in your diet is that when both are applied on your skin and taken, it would reduce the eczema attack severity.

You can treat your eczema attack quicker compared to other herbal remedies, according to research throughout the years.

Milk vetch (Astragalus Membranaeceus)

This is one of the most important plants that are used in traditional Chinese medication. It has been used for the past 2000 years to help strengthen your body. When it comes to using milk vetch to deal with eczema, the most important thing to understand is that it is an adaptogen. Adaptogen is a form of substance which helps the body to de-stress, physically and psychologically. It also helps reduce stress naturally.

A very common practice in China is to boil a piece of Astragalus root with ginseng and other health-giving plants. And then, discard the root and serve. This isn't only very nutritious, but very delicious.

The various studies on the effects of milk vetch have shown that the plant offers 'unspecific' immune system advantages. Instead of activating your body's defense mechanism against another particular form of infection, it would boost your immune system by increasing the number of macrophages. Macrophages are very important white blood cells which gives strength to your immune system and its ability to resist attack.

Besides that, milk vetch also possesses tissue regenerating and certain anti-inflammatory qualities. It gives a great deal of help to people who suffer from eczema as it reduces the inflammation and also help new healthy skin tissue to grow. It also has multiple powerful antibacterial qualities as well. Without a doubt, this is certainly an herbal remedy that you should include in your diet.

Garlic

Garlic has an active ingredient which gives a pungent smell. It is a sulphur-rich volatile oil known as allicin. This oil gives garlic that ability to boost your immune system while stimulating your blood circulation and kill bacteria. Garlic is a natural antibacterial substance which helps improve your immune system. It would strengthen your body's ability to reduce the frequency and severity of eczema.

Besides that, garlic also has multiple qualities that would boost your immune system in fighting any kinds of infections or medical conditions like eczema. As an example, garlic is known to be anti-parasitic, anti-septic, anti-viral and anti-fungal. Without a doubt, a healthy dose of garlic in your diet would give your immunity a boost, which helps to deal with eczema over the long term.

However, it should be noted that eating too much garlic each day may make your breath unpleasant. As such, many sufferers who suffer from various conditions prefer taking garlic capsule rather than including garlic in their diet. There isn't anything wrong with this, but it could be more expensive than simply including garlic into your diet. It is much easier to include garlic in your diet than having the buy a stream of garlic capsules.

Shitake Mushrooms

Shitake mushrooms have been used in many parts of Chinese medications for a few thousand years. Even now in Japan, it is used in chemotherapy and radiation to ensure that patients recover much faster. The reason why it is used so regularly is because Shitake mushrooms has the great ability of penetrating deep into the bone marrow of the person who eats it regularly.

For sufferers of eczema, it should be known that there is a certain substance in this mushroom known as lentinan. It has shown that this substance have the incredible ability to stimulate the growth of T-cells while stimulating it also increases macrophage activity. It would also boost the strength and numbers of white blood cells, which is an indication of having a strong immune system.

It should be noted that all these are very relevant in boosting your immunity as lentinan has great ability in increasing production of immune competent cells. Having Shitake mushrooms in your diet would be great to boost your immune system and it would fight back against those eczema attacks that sufferers have. This is something that you should definitely consider.

Honey

Honey is often considered a 'super-food'. It is a natural antibacterial substance because it has an ability to boost your immunity, increase your energy levels and vitality. Many people think that honey is simply something sweet that bees make, but there are a complex mix of organic acids, antibacterial agents and other minerals like copper, iron and zinc.

In the past chapters, I have mentioned that zinc is extremely important in your diet to fight eczema naturally. As such, including honey in your daily intake is a very great move. As a matter of fact, honey has other great qualities for eczema sufferers. Honey also help with surgical wound infections and skin burns.

Simply apply them on your skin to ensure a faster cure.

There has been much evidence that burns would respond better and quicker compared to pharmaceutical burn treatments. You shouldn't just include honey in your diet, but also apply it to the areas on your skin which is affected by eczema to bring instant relief to your itch and reduce the scarring.

Other Herbs

Besides the natural substances mentioned in this chapter, there are also other herbal remedies that sufferers could use to help offset the effects of eczema.

Many of those herbs should be applied to your skin which is affected by eczema, ideally after you have made a suitable oil compound with mild baby oil. Among the herbs you could use include cleavers, nettles, red clover and yellow dock leaves.

You can also use lotions which are based on chamomile and primrose oil, which have brought great relief to eczema sufferers. We have also considered how olive oil and tea tree for application as a topical eczema treatment as it has soothing qualities. It should be noted, that there isn't any fast and hard rule about what works and what don't work for an eczema sufferer. Therefore, you would need to try everything before deciding what works for you.

Final Notes

In the past few chapters, we have shared the methods of dealing with eczema naturally. It is the better alternative compared to other forms of medication. I normally recommend natural treatment first, before anything.

It is without a doubt that most medical practitioners would insist that you take pharmaceuticals like antihistamines or corticosteroids.

However, you don't have to resort to these potentially dangerous drugs unless your eczema problem becomes so bad that natural treatment is totally ineffective. Luckily, this is very unlikely. Most people who suffer from eczema will have to deal with intense itching from time to time, but it would unlikely be too dangerous.

It should be noted that there isn't an eczema experts that can claim to fully understand the condition. This condition is truly understood by scientists or researchers; and as such, it would be impossible for doctors to prescribe the 'magic medication' as well. For them to cure your eczema would be more or less impossible.

If you have spent years trying to tame your eczema problem through medication, you should try a more natural approach. However, if the natural solutions that you try don't work, you can try other alternative natural treatment. From this book alone, I have shared multiple treatments which I have found.

All of these natural treatments have proven to work but some would work far better for you than for others. To conclude, you now have plenty of natural treatments for eczema available. Start it now, to ensure that you get the best results from it. Good luck!

Resource 1 - Cure Eczema In 14 Days

Permanently CURE Eczema In 14 days!

"This Is An Eczema Cure That Is <u>Guaranteed To Get</u> You Absolutely CLEAR And BEAUTIFUL SKIN In 2 weeks!!!"

<u>Do you want to...</u>

- Get Rid of Your Severe Eczema Itching!
- *No More Scratching Endlessly!*

- No More Need to Resist the Unbearable Urge To scratch!
- *No More Hiding Your Eczema Scars!*
- Sleep Well at Night!
- *Wake Up Feeling Refreshed and Not Having To Look at The Consequences of Scratching!*
- Have Clear and Beautiful Skin Now!

If you are serious about curing your eczema problem, check out this website: http://eczema14days.wellbeingvalley.com/

Resource 2 - Beat Eczema Naturally

In this guide, you would find natural cures for eczema. The free guide from this link alone is worth gold.

This is the greatest guide that I have seen on natural cures for eczema. Check out the link for the free guide which is something that I give to everyone that I know with eczema.

Check it out at:

http://beateczema.wellbeingvalley.com/

www.ingramcontent.com/pod-product-compliance
Lightning Source LLC
Chambersburg PA
CBHW070553290526
45790CB00002B/673